HEALTHY AGEING

A guide to secrets of Healthy Ageing

International Edition

Author : Dr Neeraj Kaushik

Co-author: Dr Manika Kaushik

Contents

Introduction

In Indian yoga there is an old saying that die young but as late as possible.   Many people may not know that we are now living in the 'Decade of Healthy Ageing', as declared by the United Nations General Assembly in 2020. Healthy ageing which has the potential to increase not only life expectancy but overall health and wellbeing of an aged person. There are many human races in various parts of the world that are healthy despite of ageing. I know a heart surgeon who was doing cardiac surgeries at an age of hundred years, a ninety year old couple walking uphill without getting tired, a man of eighty four years running every day, my own grandmother who never had any health issue, a ninety year old man doing Tai Chi for hours, a ninety plus year yoga teacher practicing and teaching yoga to the world and so on. This brings me to think why some people are healthy at such an old stage and why age related diseases are not bothering them, why no dementia, no joint problems, no infections, no heart, lung and BP problems.

The purpose of writing this book is to help you understand human ageing process and what action can be taken to avoid or minimize the impact of ageing on your health so that you can lead a healthy and dignified life totally independent and without depending on others. A healthy happy life when you age is possible and this book is here to train you for that. It will cover areas to understand ageing and various tools and techniques including Ayurveda, Chinese Medicine, Japanese Ikegai, Mediterranean diet and role of nature in health and wellness. This book explains the role of various techniques in reversing your age related health issues like diabetes, hypertension, infections, immunity issues, dementia, and joint problems.

The aim of writing this book is to help you live a healthy and quality life with least dependence on drugs and medical care.

Positive Ageing

The Australian Psychological Society defines positive ageing as "the process of maintaining a positive attitude, feeling good about yourself, keeping fit and healthy, and engaging fully in life as you age". Ageing is a natural process which everyone faces during his or her life cycle. The bad news is that ageing brings in many age related diseases making life dependent of drugs and others and the good news is that most of them are preventable and manageable. The concept of positive and healthy ageing focuses on maintaining a growth mindset or ikigai as the Japanese follow in their life to live a better and healthier life especially in the old age. Age is just a number if you have a positive ageing attitude.

Research have shown that a positive attitude towards life improves physical and mental health and enables older people to retain their control and quality of life and can live longer. Although many aspects of health are genetic but there are many facets of health and aging are within our control. Ageing has got its own health challenges but with a positive attitude you can keep them in control to enjoy a healthy and quality life.

Although we are partially limited by our genetics in our ability to age healthily, our physical and social environments still play a significant role. We should be able act to change these factors of ageing or improve them with time.

Tips for Positive aging:

Maintain an active life style but avoid overdoing, know your limits.

Sitting is new smoking and increases stiffness, tightness and pain & can take away many years from your life. As we move older, we stop moving our body. Even if you are 20 year old and stop moving your body, you get the same thing, ageing, stiffness, pain, body degeneration and blockages. Movement is the key to health & longevity.

Exercise at least five days a week. Exercise makes you less prone to diseases, improves appearance, delays aging, and reduces chances of lifestyle diseases including heart diseases, diabetes, high BP etc. Regular and repeated exercise on daily basis is the key to good health as exercises keep your muscles and body shape intact as well as strengthen you sympathetic and parasympathetic nervous system which help you in age slow. Now what is exercise and how to do it? Walking, yoga, moving all the joints to keep them active and healthy, climbing, Qi-gong, Tia Chi, dancing, are all forms of exercise.

Keep the child in you alive. Do not over think and keep the child in you alive. As ageing leads to anxiety, fear, depression and loneliness, keep the child inside you active. A child is fearless, happy, no anxiety and no thinking of past and future. Be one and do not care what will happen in future, live in the present. No burden of past memories and no fear of future.

Change your diet pattern. Your food become medicine, switch to healthy and natural food and food that heals the body and delays ageing. Try to eat homemade or self-made food where you are well aware what is inside and which ingredients are used to prepare it.

Go for community living. Research proves that people who live in communities live healthy and long as the community living help in reducing stress levels and improving happiness level.

Always be ready to help others. Having a helping attitude and helping others will boost the flow of happy and healthy hormones and your confidence level will be up. Whenever you get an opportunity do it and if possible indulge yourself in some charitable activity.

Diet & Ageing

Wrong diet choices result in faster ageing process. Unhealthy diets along with physical inactivity are the major risk factors for chronic diseases which pose threat in older age. First of all, you should set up a goal for nutrient intake in order to prevent age related chronic disorders.

What to include in your diet?

Fruits, vegetables, nuts and whole grains like unprocessed maize, brown rice, oats, millet and organic wheat must become integral part of your daily diet. Your per day intake may be around 400 grams. Sugar intake should not come from processed sugar. Whatever sugar is added to food can be naturally sugar which is naturally present in honey, fruit juices but in any case you should take less than 10% of your energy intake from sugar.

When it comes to the consumption of fats, it should come from unsaturated fat found in olive oil, nuts, seeds, avocado & fish. Minimize the use of saturated fats which is available in coconut oil, cheese, butter. Put a strict ban on trans-fat found in processed & fast food as the trans-fat is really bad for your healthy ageing. Also limit the use of salt in your diet. Try to restrict the salt usage around 5 gram a day as salt contains sodium element which is responsible for high blood pressure and water accumulation in the body leading to many life threatening issued especially in the older age.

When you include, around 400 grams of fruits and vegetables every day in your diet, you are actually reducing the chances of age related chronic diseases significantly and it also nourished you with sufficient dietary fibers. Dietary fiber is very important part of a good digestive system and keeps your problem like Diabetes, high blood pressure, constipation in check.

Nutrition

Nutrition is an important part of health and development and a good nutrition help in maintaining age related diseases under control, improved physical and mental health, strong immune system and longevity. Today ageing population is falling sick not because of the mal-nutrition but eating in excess. So now days, most of the diseases are excessive diseases. Your aim should be a good and adequate nutrition depending on body's dietary needs. The best formula for healthy ageing is balanced diet combined with regular physical activity. Bad diet choice can lead to reduced immunity and increased chance of infection, poor mental and physical development.

In the 21st century, nutrition has become more focused on how diseases, health condition and problems can be prevented or reduced with the healthy diet for a healthy ageing. A good nutrition help in identifying how age related diseases can be prevented or reversed for ensuring a good health. In India, traditional Indian medicine always believes to have food as medicine with the aim of a good health.

Types of Nutrients

A nutrient is a component of food and comprises of:

- Carbohydrates

- Fats

- Proteins

- Vitamins

- Minerals

- Water

Carbohydrates, fats and proteins are also known as macro nutrients which provide energy and are the basic building blocks of the body. Body needs them in large quantities. A macro nutrient that does not provide energy but still needed in large quantity includes water and fiber.

Carbohydrates:
They are energy giving macro nutrient and provide Four Kcal per gram. They are divided into Monosaccharide, Disaccharides and poly-saccharides. Poly-saccharides are favored as they are more complex and do not break down easily, have lot of fiber and hardly cause spike in blood sugar level which is one of the cause of Diabetes.

Fats:

Fats are important macro nutrient and contain Nine Kcal per gram. They are required for many body functions including brain health, hormone production, reducing body inflammation, absorption of certain vitamins and joint lubrication and giving you energy when you require it in large amount.

Proteins:

These categories of macronutrients are the building blocks of body and your body shape, muscle mass and in fact immunity is decided by them. One gram of protein gives four Kcal of energy. Proteins are basically made up of amino acids that combine to form the protein structure. There are two categories of proteins: essential and non-essential. Non-essential amino acids can be made by body but essential amino acids needs to be consumed. Consumption of proteins adequate amount of protein is required to maintain your body shape and muscle mass especially in the aged people. There are many sources of proteins which include vegetable like broccoli and other green leafy vegetables, meat, pulses, milk and milk products.

In Indian vegetarian diet, there are very good combination of protein like kidney beans (Rajma) and other pulses along with Rice, millets and legume combination.

Other Macro Nutrients

Fiber:

Dietary fibers are non-starch poly saccharides carbohydrate and other plant component which help in lowering blood sugar level, reducing bad cholesterol level and prevent colon cancer. With a healthy ageing, always keep in mind intake of fibrous food.

Water:
Our body and every cell have 72% water. For taking care of your health it is very essential that you drink plenty of water. Drink small amount of water frequently may be around 250 ml every hour. Electrolyte plays a very important role in water retention. Replace lost electrolyte immediately. Take some foods that have high water content and very low in calories like watermelon, pineapple, strawberry, orange and celery. Water help in your body detox and if you drink water as first drink in the morning, it triggers gastro colic reflex which stimulates bowel movement. Avoid water for at least 45 minutes after meals. This will help in better and fast digestion of food.

Micronutrients: Minerals

Calcium – is one of the most important micro nutrient required by our body. It has many important functions like building bones, assisting in synthesis and functions of blood cells, muscle health, heart health, digestive health and in fact health of the thyroid gland. It starts depleting from our bones after thirty years of age and keeping a regular check on the calcium level is important. Regular intake of Calcium either as supplement or through food containing calcium like milk and milk products, raagi etc. is important especially in the old age to maintain a good health and a firm body shape.

Sodium and Potassium – this are systemic electrolytes and essential in regulating normal blood pressure as well as ATP. Potassium is also important for nerve functions as well as regulating body fluids.

Phosphorus – it is important for our DNA and is transporter of energy i.e. ATP. It is also helpful in strengthening bones especially during old age.

Chloride – it is important micro nutrient for stomach acid and vital for proper functioning of nerves.

Iron – the most part of the hemoglobin of the blood and it also required for proteins and other enzymes.

Zinc – it is one of the most important micro nutrients for anti-ageing. It is important for reproductive organ growth, many genes and enzymes, proper nerve functioning as well as good immunity in the old age.

Magnesium – required for the energy of the body as well as bones and muscles. It is also an important part of enzymes of the body along with manganese and copper.

Iodine – required for biosynthesis of thyroxine, an important hormone for body metabolism.

Selenium – it is an important micro nutrient for taking care of free radicals which accumulates and damages your DNA and age you fast as it is also required for anti-oxidant enzymes and delays ageing.

Molybdenum – it has vital role in carbohydrate metabolism, body detoxification and uric acid formation.

Vitamins

Vitamins are essential micro nutrient without which survival is not possible and for a healthy ageing a proper balance of vitamins in the body is crucial. There are two categories of the vitamins found in the body out of which four are fat soluble vitamin like A,D, E and K which are accumulated in the body and stored. The other category of vitamins is nine water soluble vitamins where eight are part of the B complex and ninth is vitamin C.

Every vitamin has got a different function in the body and is responsible for the complete body metabolism. Deficiency of these vitamins can cause many diseases and are their adequate quantity must be balanced through regular intake of this second category of vitamins. This category of vitamin is water soluble and cannot be stored in the body. One precaution you have to take that if you are taking vitamin supplement, make sure that there is no overdose of any vitamin as it can do more harm than good. The best source of vitamins is not pill but your seasonable fruits and vegetables.

Physical activity

Sitting is new smoking and increases stiffness, tightness and pain & can take away many years from your life.

As we move older, we stop moving our body. Even if you are 20 year old and stop moving your body, you get the same thing, ageing, stiffness, pain, body degeneration and blockages.

MOVEMENT IS THE KEY TO HEALTH AND LONGEVITY.

Exercise makes you less prone to diseases, improves appearance, delays ageing, reduce chances of lifestyle diseases including heart diseases, diabetes, high BP etc.

Physical inactivity is one of the leading risk factors for age related problems and can age you fast. Regular moderate physical activity like walking, cycling, dancing, playing, yoga, tai-chi, qi-gong can have significant benefit for your health and has the potential to delay ageing and keep you fit in your old age. Adequate levels of physical activity will decrease the risk of cardio vascular diseases, dementia, fractures, diabetes, depression and many kinds of cancer related to ageing. You should do at least 150 minutes of moderate physical activity throughout the week to remain yourself in balance and in shape.

Muscle strengthening exercises should be done for at least three days a week along with the regular physical activity. The physical activity is actually any bodily movement produced by skeletal muscles that requires energy expenditure. Physical activity includes working, playing, carrying out household chores, travelling and engaging in recreational activity.

Misconceptions on Ageing and Health

Older people are care dependent.

No they are not. Statistics proves that only a small proportion of older people are care dependent. Older people in fact make major contribution to families and society.

Older people are having diseases and are inactive because of that.

Again it's a myth. Older people despite of having some health conditions are living independently and contributing to society as a whole. It is the combination of physical and mental capabilities which is better indicator of health and wellbeing rather than presence of certain disease.

Genetic factors

Although genetics play a role and healthy ageing starts at birth but that contributes to 25% in determining longevity. The other 75% is largely the result of our physical and social environment and our lifestyle.

Common Health Problems associated with Ageing

Old age has some health issues but as per WHO most of them are preventable and manageable. Common health problems in the old age includes frequent infection, depression, dementia, heart problem, pulmonary disease, joint pain especially neck, back & knee pain, osteoarthritis, hearing loss, high blood pressure and diabetes. All these problems can be minimized or dealt with by maintaining a healthy and active lifestyle during the old age. These problems along with others can be tackled by adopting healthy behavior, eating a balance diet, engaging in regular physical activity, improving physical and mental capacity, strengthening training to maintain muscle mass, good nutrition are the tools for a healthy ageing.

Ageing & Heart Disease

Managing heart health with ageing is absolutely crucial for longevity and quality of life. The human body is one of the best machines in the universe and if maintained properly, it can't develop a snag. 95% of the heart diseases can be prevented or even reversed with the help of education & knowledge about it and taking basic necessary action yourself.

Coronary Artery Disease (CAD) which is the main heart issue can be also be called as the disease of ignorance & is a result of long term mismanagement of heart health with stress, wrong diet, sedentary lifestyle & smoking.

Personality and environment play a big role in heart disease. A potential heart patient is in hurry all the time with lack of patience, has a perfectionist and not a practical attitude, restlessness, always preoccupied mind, excessively critical of self & others, gets provoked easily, highly dominating, always stressed. Apart from these personality attributes, the potential heart patient lives a sedentary lifestyle with either very less or lack of physical exercise, his/her dietary habits & choice of food is also unhealthy & above all he/she is not educated or aware of the heart & its health.

Are you at risk for heart disease or stroke?

The good news is that almost 80% of premature heart disease and stroke can be prevented through healthy lifestyle habits. Knowing your own risk factors is the first step to help prevent disease.

Assess your risk

Learn how to reduce your risk

Take action

First step is to assess your risk.

Check the risk factors that apply to you.

Medical conditions

- High blood pressure
- High cholesterol
- Diabetes
- Sleep apnea (a condition that causes you to stop and start breathing while you sleep)

Lifestyle risk factors

- Unhealthy diet
- Not enough exercise
- Obesity
- Smoking, Tobacco use
- Heavy drinking
- Stress

Risk factors you cannot control

- Age (the older you are, the higher your risk)
- Sex (your risk of heart disease and stroke increases with menopause)
- Family history of heart disease, stroke or ischemic attack

Step 2 Learn how to reduce your risk

Manage your medical conditions

High blood pressure is the number one risk factor for stroke and a major risk factor for heart disease. You cannot feel or notice high blood pressure. The only way to know if you have high blood pressure is to measure it.

Take Action

- Ask your doctor for your target blood pressure level. Check it regularly.
- Take medication, if prescribed by your doctor.
- Reduce the amount of salt you eat. Specially take note of the sodium intake.
- Eat a healthy balanced diet, with lots of vegetables and fruit.
- Try to stay at a healthy weight. BMI less than 25. Learn healthy diet.

- Be more active. Keep Moving and avoid long sitting.
- Be smoke free.
- Manage stress.

Improve cholesterol levels

High blood cholesterol is one of the major controllable risk factors for heart disease and stroke. As your blood cholesterol rises, so does your risk of coronary heart disease.

Take Action

- Eat a healthy balanced diet, with lots of vegetables and fruit.
- Be smoke-free.
- Try to stay at a healthy weight.
- Be more active.
- Take medication, if prescribed by your doctor.

Control diabetes

People with diabetes are three times more likely to have heart disease. They are also more likely to develop heart disease at a younger age.

Take Action

- HbA1C - Monitor and control your blood sugar levels.
- Blood pressure - Know your blood pressure and take steps to keep it in a healthy range.
- Cholesterol - Make sure your LDL cholesterol levels are low.
- Drugs to decrease heart disease risk. This might include blood pressure pills, cholesterol-lowering pills and others.
- Exercise and healthy eating.
- Self-management support. Set goals to reach and maintain a healthy lifestyle and understand what stands in your way.
- Screening or monitoring for complications.
- Stop smoking.

Make lifestyle changes to improve your health

Eat healthy

You can improve your heart and brain health by eating a healthy balanced diet.

Take Action

- Eat a healthy balanced diet, with lots of vegetables and fruit.
    - Choose brightly colored fruits and vegetables each day, especially orange and dark green vegetables.
    - Frozen or canned unsweetened fruits and vegetables are a good alternative to fresh produce.
- Prepare meals at home from scratch. Cooking at home allows you to select whole and minimally processed foods, and to limit added salt.
- Keep a reusable water bottle with you so that you can fill it up wherever you are going. Communities that do not have access to safe drinking water can stay hydrated with non-sweetened drinks such as coffee, tea or boiled water.

Be physically more active

Being physically active is good for your heart and brain. Getting 150 minutes of moderate to vigorous-intensity activity per week can significantly reduce the risk of heart disease, stroke, high blood pressure and diabetes. People who are NOT active have an increased risk of heart disease and stroke, as well as an increased risk of diabetes, cancer and dementia. Being active helps your heart, brain, muscles, bones and mood.

Take Action

- Try to be active every day. — Aim for 30 minutes of physical activity most days of the week, in sessions of 10 minutes or more.
    - Include moderate exercise (cycling, brisk walking, jogging) in the mix.
- Walking is a great way to start.
- Look for opportunities to be active every day. Play outside with the kids, take leaves, take the stairs...it is all good!
- Start slowly, set weekly goals and increase your level of activity over time.

Aim for a healthy weight

Being overweight can lead to high blood pressure, high cholesterol, diabetes and sleep apnea. Even a small weight loss will help.

Take Action

- Your doctor will help you figure out the weight that is right for you.
- The best way to lose weight is to choose healthy food and be more active.
- Make small changes in your diet and activity levels that you can keep for life. That's better than making lots of changes at once and not sticking to any of them.

Kick the smoking habit

Smokers have more than twice the risk for heart attack. Smoking triples the risk of dying from heart disease and stroke in middle-aged men and women. Quitting is one of the most important things you can do to prevent heart disease and stroke.

Drink less alcohol

Heavy drinking and binge drinking are risk factors for heart disease and stroke. Plus, alcohol may cause problems by interacting with your medications.

Take Action

- If you drink alcohol, drink in moderation.

Manage stress

Stress can cause the heart to work harder, increases blood pressure and increases your risk.

Take Action

- Know what causes you stress.
- Talk to people you trust.
- Take a short break away from your regular routine.
- Plan some physical activity into your day.
- Try mindfulness meditation or deep breathing to help you relax.
- Do activities you enjoy. Have some fun!

Step 3 Take Action
Make changes for a healthier life

• Plan to make healthy lifestyle changes that include realistic goals — like walking for 20 minutes, 5 days a week. Ask yourself how confident you are about reaching the goal. If you don't feel confident, change the goal to one you can reach.

• Act on your goals — take one step at a time.

• Figure out what's stopping you from sticking to your plan. Keep a record of your daily food intake and physical activity to help you identify barriers and inspire you to reach your goals.

• Don't give up — get back on track when you slip up.
• Reward yourself for the gains you've made — with something you like to do, not food.

Secrets of Healthy aging & longevity

Japanese Secret: Japanese people are known for healthy and long life and this comes true when a study was conducted in Okinawa, Japan, where people live above 100 years. Secret of Okinawa residents for a healthy and long life:

- Breathe in, breathe out exercises is their daily routine

- Light physical exercises and keep themselves active

- DHEA produced by adrenal: In Okinawans levels of DHEA (youth hormone) declines very slowly as they are active people, happy people, live in community, stress free

- Fruits & vegetables dependence including dark green, yellow & red vegetables & sweet potatoes. They grow vegetables and fruits and their major diet is the same.

- High quantity of soya proteins. Okinawans have lowest rate of cancers because of soya.

- Controlled starvation – they do not over eat. Fill 80% belly & never full stomach or over eating. This controlled starvation keeps them young.

- They only eat raw food or homemade food. Never eat outside in hotels.

Mediterranean People's longevity secrets

- Genetically healthy

- In a community in Lomelinda, California, a 92 years old doctor was found doing open heart surgery successfully.

- Daily routine of a 102 years lady does following :

- cycling 6 miles before breakfast
- Exercises & meditate. By exercising & meditation a faith is developed in you to live longer & live healthy.
- Making choices & defeating fundamental forces of aging

- Do not drink & smoke

- Vegetarian diet

- They believe to live longer & they live longer

- Faith/religion/spiritual

- Religion reduces stress & delay aging.

- These people have low levels of stress hormones like cortisones & better equipped to take on life shocks.

- Try not to take life too seriously & live an easy life.

- Community living

- Laughing reduces aging

A 102 years old Okinawan man says: I hardly get angry & I enjoy life as I enjoy my work

- They think themselves young & practice Karate at 80 & 90

- They have positive & hopeful attitude

- They have simple life style

- They want to remain healthy & they are healthy

- Keep active by working in fields & sports & develops psychological resilience

- Adopt traditional diet – low fat, high calcium, similar to Atkins's diet, dark vegetables, sweet potato

- Live disciplined life

PEOPLE OF HUNZA VALLEY

- They live 100 plus with zero incidence of heart disease and cancer.

- Consume plant and raw food.

- Mainly fruits, vegetables, cereals, cheese.

- In winter dried apricot, sheep cheese, and sprouted cereals.

- For 3 months, they do not eat anything but drink only dried apricot juice.

- Hunza's are happy and good mood people.

- Hunzas are physically very active.

- Hunzas are vegetarians, eat lot of raw food generally fruits and vegetables.

- They observe starvation period of minimum one month.

Japanese holds the secret to live long

The Japanese life expectancy is the world's highest, at 87.32 years for women and 81.25 years for men. We dive into Japan's top secrets to good health and longevity.

Japanese diet is balanced, with staple foods like omega-rich fish, rice, whole grains, tofu, soy, seaweed and vegetables. All these foods are low in saturated fats and sugars and rich in vitamins and minerals that reduce the risk of cancers and heart disease. One of the oldest lady of Kagoshima, Japan shares her secret which is good sleep, moderate activities and 3 small meals. One of the major reasons is that Japanese not only eat healthy but eat less. Japanese train their young generation by developing healthy eating activities starting from primary school level with focus on lunches with plenty of fruits and vegetables. This habit lasts till Japanese whole life span.

Japanese lead an active lifestyle and not the sedentary one and this active lifestyle is imbibed at a very young age. Most of the Japanese children go to school walking or cycling. Government also promotes such activities with the help of radio and other media. Most people prefer walking or cycling to the train station, prefer standing on the train, then walk down to office.

Japan has one of the best healthcare systems in the world with special focus on preventive healthcare by facilitating healthcare scanning at school, corporate and community levels.

Ikigai is also an important tool which help Japanese keep themselves healthy and worthy. And it is proven medically that Ikigai is helpful in healthy and long life.

Ikigai is 'reason for being. Ikigai is a Japanese concept that means your 'reason for being. ' 'Iki' in Japanese means 'life,' and 'gai' describes value or worth. Your ikigai is your life purpose or your bliss. It's what brings you joy and inspires you to get out of bed every day.

Basic rules of Ikigai include:

1. Stay active; don't retire. Keep the purpose of life, do not retire and keep doing work you love irrespective of age. It will give you purpose of life to grow and keep growing. This will keep good hormones in your body intact which slowdown aging.

2. Take it slow, don't be in a hurry. Walk slowly and you'll go far. If you hurry, you will remain stressed which means more stress hormones like cortisol, more inflammation, less immunity and faster aging.

3. Don't fill your stomach. Keep 20% empty. Whether it's Ayurveda, Chinese medicine, or Japanese traditional health system, do never fill your stomach completely, eat less and live more.

4. Surround yourself with good friends and live in community "Friends are the best medicine as they are the best stress buster. Your stress level is reduced significantly, if you live in community and have lot of friends. Have fun, laugh, behave like child, dream and above all be always ready to help others. Helping others give you the best feeling and a purpose in life, share your stories with friends, listen their stories, in other words live a light and tension free life.

5. Maintain your health with active lifestyle and moderate exercise
Sedentary lifestyle is the root cause of 80% life threatening diseases, be active and do moderate exercises to keep you in shape.

6. Smile
It cost nothing to smile but can keep you young and healthy, so keep smiling so that all the good and healthy hormones can remain in good quantity in your blood to keep you happy and healthy.

7. Live with nature

The more you go away from nature, the more you will be sick and unhealthy. Follow the nature's rules for healthy and long life. Japanese use shinrin-yoku (forest bathing) which means connect with nature using the five senses of sight, hearing, taste, smell, and touch. It is a mindfulness practice to help you reconnect with nature so that you can rejuvenate the body and give the mind a moment of peace and give your body what is needs.

8. Show attitude of gratitude.
Always thank by showing attitude of gratitude to your parents, friends, co-workers, family who were always there with you to make you feel happy and healthy.

9. Live in the moment
All philosophies of the world come to one simple conclusion for a stress free happy life and that is live in the present moment. It helps you in removing burden of the past and tensions of the future. "Stop regretting the past and fearing the future. Today is all you have. Make the most of it. Make it worth remembering."

10. Always be ready to help others. Helping other will boost rush of happy or anti-ageing hormones.

11. Follow your ikigai
Always believe and follow you Ikigai means purpose of life, make your life worth.

Apart from all this Japanese also enjoy good genes which help them keeping healthy.

Meditation is the secret of good health

Meditation is conscious withdrawal from thought world. In meditation you are not karta (doer) but you are simply an observer. In meditation silence of senses illuminates the presence of higher self within. Meditation is an effort in the beginning, later on it becomes a habit and gives bliss, joy, peace and a good health.

In meditation process, fetters are undone, internal blocks of suffering such as fear, anger, despair and hatred get removed and there is freedom from thoughts and joy.

Meditation posture

 Step 1: Sit in any posture which is comfortable for you. You can choose to sit on floor or on a chair.

Step 2: Cross your legs, clasp your fingers and sit comfortably.

Step 3: Close your eyes, stop inner or outer chatter. Do not chant any mantra, just relax, and totally relax. When your fingers are clasped and legs crossed, energy circles develop around you to give stability. Eyes are doors to the mind so for better meditation experience, it is better to keep the eyes closed. Mantra chanting or any other thoughts and activities of mind should be stopped.

Step 4: When body relaxes, consciousness travels to next door which is mind and intellect. As mind is full of thoughts, to transcend the mind & intellect, one has to observe the breath. Just focus your attention on natural breathing. Just observe, do not force.

Step 5: Observation is the witness of self, so just observe the breath, no conscious breathing, just observes the natural breathing.

THIS IS THE KEY.

Do not go behind thoughts, observe normal breathing, and be with your breath. As you keep focusing on your breath, the density of thoughts reduces and slowly breath becomes thinner and shorter. Finally breath becomes smallest and settles like a flash in between the eyebrows, in this state one will have no breath and no thought. You will become completely thoughtless. This state is called meditative state or thoughtless state. In this state your mind's healing power is thousand times the normal one and according to Indian Yog, you will be under the shower of cosmic energy. More meditation, more cosmic energy. This cosmic energy flows throughout the body called Etheric body that means all your chakras or energy centers are under the shower of this energy.

Sleep is unconscious meditation while meditation is conscious sleep. During sleep we get limited energy while during meditation we get abundant energy. This energy enhances power of our body, mind, and intellect. It opens the door for our sixth sense and beyond. In meditation, we travel from body to mind to intellect to self and beyond.

CHAKRA MEDITATION

Chakras are energy centers that unite mind, body and spirit. There are seven energy centers in human body and meditating on these chakras has immense health benefits. Chakras process and distribute energy that is needed for our health, well-being and vitality,

Root Chakra (Muladhar)

Located at the base of your spine, this chakra's energetic function is to help us maintain physical health including body strength. Root Chakra has 4 lotus shape petals red in color. Meditate on this chakra and visualize these red petals are opening and shining more and more.

Sacral Chakra (Svadhisthana)

Located at your pelvis, this chakra's energetic function is to help us regulate our emotions and desires, so as not to be driven by them. It has 6 orange color lotus shaped petals. Meditate on this chakra and visualize these petals are opening and shining more and more.

Solar Plexus Chakra (Manipura)
Located at your belly button, this chakra gives us the confidence we need to process and eliminate what does not serve us, and to let it go.

It has 10 yellow color lotus shaped petals. Meditate on this chakra and visualize these petals are opening and shining more and more.

Heart Chakra (Anahata)
Located at the center of your chest, this chakra's energetic function is to help us tap into unconditional love. It has 12 green color lotus shaped petals. Meditate on this chakra and visualize these petals are opening and shining more and more.

Throat Chakra (Vishuddha)
Located at the base of your throat, this chakra's energetic function is to help us find authentic self-expression. . It has 16 light blue color lotus shaped petals. Meditate on this chakra and visualize these petals are opening and shining more and more.

Third Eye Chakra (Ajna)
Located on your forehead in between your eyes, this chakra's energetic function is to help us learn to know ourselves emotionally, mentally and spiritually. It has 2 navy blue color lotus shaped petals. Meditate on this chakra and visualize these petals are opening and shining more and more.

Crown Chakra (Sahasrara)
Located at the top of the head, this chakra helps us function in a more enlightened way, cultivate self-mastery and find a sense of connection with all. It has 1000 violet color lotus shaped petals. Meditate on this chakra and visualize these petals are opening and shining more and more.

SOHUM MEDITATION

Sohum is mahamantra and is one of the most ancient type of meditation. Sohum is sound of breathing. Sound of inhalation is SO and sound of exhalation is HUM. If you combine both it becomes SOHUM. SOHUM means I am HE higher self), so you are calling higher self, every breath becomes a prayer and adoration.

Technique:
Sit in a comfortable posture and relax. Close your eyes and ears, command mind to be silent and calm, relax your body with no tension on any muscle, just relax. A very light meditational instrumental music at the background is ok.

Focus on sound of breath. While inhalation observe sound SO and during exhalation observe sound HUM. Keep repeating this for 20 minutes. Observe one breath after another, feel how we are rewarded with one breath after another.

NON EXPRESSION OF NEGATIVITY Meditation

Practice in your daily routine not to say or think anything negative, either be positive or neutral.

AUM or OM Meditation

OM is a universal sound energy. It is within everyone and everything. When you chant OM, all universal energies and their vibrations connect with you. With practice, your energy merges with universal energies and you receive healing energies. Om meditation controls your breath with more involvement of parasympathetic nervous system, decreasing your blood pressure and balances your body, mind and intellect.
Technique: Sit in a comfortable position and relax whole body. Breathe in to full capacity and while exhaling chant OM slowly and deeply, exhale deep and completely with OM, the more time you take for exhalation, the better it will be.

Do it for 20 minutes and you will feel relaxed with feeling of joy, more energetic and stiffness and tensions in muscles gone with relief in pain.

CELLULAR HEALING Meditation

Nature has given all of us a great power of healing. Healing starts the moment we bring our mind's attention to that place. Healing starts the moment we believe it will occur. The moment your mind buys into it, your body makes it happen.
Procedure:
Sit comfortably and relax body and mind with few deep breathings and close your eyes. Now focus and see from your mind's eye the following:
- Watch damage cells changing into healthy cells and becoming free from injuries. Visualize all cells as completely healthy. Maintain natural breathing.

- Watch your protector cells within your body attacking and killing damaged or infected cells and replacing these diseased cells with the normal ones.
- Your defensive cell eating all threatening cells and your body is free of dangerous cells. Visualize groups of healthy cells combining and replacing damaged cells of the body. Visualize healing energies filling you.
- While inhaling, visualize healing air flowing through lungs to all the cells and removing pain and stiffness. If you sincerely wish healing to take place, believe in it.

This is a good meditation technique, which have compromised immunity and fall sick easily. This meditation technique is useful for cancer patients and patients suffering from severe infections.

PAIN HEALING Meditation

Procedure:
- Sit comfortably, relax your mind and body. Take few deep breaths with focus on breathing.
- Visualize your body is slowly filling with light, starting from feet and slowly moving upwards, relaxing and healing everything coming its way.
- Visualize diseased or painful areas as dark circles and your body of light is radiating light from your eyes like a torch. Direct this light from your eyes towards dark circles represented by disease or pain and they are healed and removed.
- Affirmation to say quietly: I radiate this light to my body to heal. And after healing my body and mind, I radiate this light to the whole world. I am radiating this healing light from my body to my room to my city to my country to the whole world. Let the whole world be healed with this healing light.
- This light is blessing me with health and vitality. Perfect health is available to me now.

OUT OF THE BODY Meditation:

- Sit comfortably, relax your mind and body. Take few deep breaths with focus on breathing.

- Visualize stepping out of body and feel being above the body looking down to self. From here, radiate and send a golden healing light to your own body.
- Focus and radiate this golden light to your body, healing all parts with rejuvenation and positive feeling. This light is detoxifying my body and cleansing away toxins including toxin thoughts. Affirm: I am healthy and happy.
- Now focus this light to heart and arteries for healthy circulatory system.
- Radiate this light energy to abdomen area, now this light is absorbed in the body and becomes energy. From here the whole body is filled with energy and healing every part of it.
- Now radiate blue light to your body and visualize blue and golden light all over the body. With this golden and blue light all over the body, say this affirmation silently: I show my gratitude to you as you are the chariot of my soul. I heal you and these golden and blue lights will take away all negative energies and remove all toxins making you pure and healthy.

UNLOCKING THE THIRD EYE Meditation

Indian Traditional Yog has given importance to the third eye and meditating on the third eye for health.
We have two eyes which are part of the physical body. There is an energy center in between the two eye brows which is also known as third eye. This is a point where you can focus and meditate and with practice this energy center becomes activated and at this point your body stops giving orders to you and instead it starts to obey your orders. Such person becomes the master of his body, mind and senses. The more you concentrate on this point and remember this center, the more you become master of yourself.
Attention is food for third eye, pay attention to it and it becomes activated with enhanced healing power of the body.

Principles to follow for better results in meditation practice:
- Visualize universal energy everywhere.
- Be non-reactive
- Be non-judgmental
- Either be positive or neutral to all
- Live in present moment
- Be non-logical
- Un-conditional love

Good Immunity means Good Health

Immunity is your answer to all the germs including bacteria and viruses. Health is not just the absence of germs, toxins, or cancer cells but it's how well your body responds to them. Good immunity means good health. Medically Immunity is a complex biological system that can recognize and tolerate whatever belongs to the self, and to recognize and reject what is foreign (non-self).

What we can do to improve immunity so that our body can fight infections well including corona. Immunity is directly linked with our lifestyle, the more we live near to nature, better is immunity and the more we live sedentary lifestyle, immunity is less so is our power to fight infections.

Simple steps for good immunity:

Avoid canned and processed foods

Canned and processed foods usually contain lots of chemical preservatives and substances that interfere with the immune system. Even if you are compelled to purchase them look at the ingredients minutely and choose the product with minimum preservatives or without preservative or artificial things.

Use Coconut oil

Coconut oil is rich in lauric and caprylic acids, the substances have antiviral and antibacterial properties.

Dark leafy greens

They contain antioxidants which are crucial for keeping the immune system healthy. They're rich in vitamins A, B6 and B12, which help fight against infections.

Nuts

Rich in vitamin E, these help fight against the decrease in immunological activity. In this group you can find almonds, chestnuts, walnuts, seeds.

Avoid stress

Stress and anxiety cause the body to release hormones including cortisols known for their immunosuppressive activity (which decreases your immune system's functionality). And you become prone to infections.

Get some sun in the morning

Vitamin D is very important for a better immune system and is easily available from sun exposure. Sunbathing helps the production of vitamin D and improves cognitive function when it comes to pregnancy and child development.

Do everything in moderation

Excess doesn't help to strengthen your immune system. This includes; overeating, alcohol consumption, drugs, cigarettes, too much physical exercise, or sleepless nights.

Avoid Excessive medication

Some medicines or drugs decrease the production of immune system cells and antibodies. Unnecessary antibiotics can also increase the resistance of bacteria resulting in compromised immunity. So avoid excessive medication for a better immune response.

Sleep well 7 to 8 hours a day

Lack of sleep can increase the body's stress levels and decrease immunity. It's recommended to sleep 7 to 8 hours per night.

Regular exercise is a must

Around 150 minutes of exercise per week is important for a good immune system. In addition to reducing stress levels and improving overall body health, exercise produces a sense of well-being that strengthens the immune system.

Golden Milk

Ayurveda has given importance to golden milk or turmeric milk in its system of medicine. This help in reducing body inflammation and is natural pain killer. It is rich in antioxidants. It is anti-inflammatory, anti-microbial, fights bacterial as well as viral infections.

Drum stick (Moringa)

Drum sticks is recommended for boosting immunity against several viruses, mainly against colds.

Ginseng

Ginseng is used worldwide for immunity and anti-ageing properties.

Onion and Garlic

It has quercetin, an immune system booster. In addition to preventing viral diseases, it's also effective in fighting allergies.

It's a source of allicin, a substance that stimulates the immune response. It's also rich in selenium and zinc, which are nutrients that help to prevent the flu and other diseases.

Citrus fruit

With a high concentration of vitamin C, these fruits increase the production of white blood cells, which are the immune cells that fight viral diseases like the flu.

Water

72% of body is water, so keep replenishing your body with adequate water. The recommendation is to drink at least 2.5 to 3 liters per day to keep hydrated.

Some Ayurvedic tips can be easily incorporated in our daily routine to boost immunity

- Avoid simple sugars in any form

- Limit alcohol,

- Avoid processed foods, microwaved foods, canned foods and foods with preservatives.

- Never drink ice water.

- Always include spices into cooking, such as turmeric, black pepper, cumin, coriander.

- Sip hot water or fresh ginger tea throughout the day to boost the digestion.

- Use clarified butter (ghee) for cooking.

- Do not overcook your food.

- Eat on fixed timings every day ant fixed intervals.

- Fast one day a week, if possible.

Dr Kaushik's Recommendation for back pain

Chronic or long-term back pain can be challenging for doctors to treat. However, it is possible to treat back pain without surgery with the help of alternative treatments such as having spinal manipulation, acupuncture, and making lifestyle changes.

Back pain is a widespread problem, with low back pain affecting most of the adults at some point in their lives. The pain may develop suddenly as a result of a muscle strain caused by heavy lifting or an accident. Other times, conditions such as arthritis, osteoporosis or scoliosis can cause back pain.

Non Surgical treatments for Back Pain

1. Chiropractic (Spinal manipulation)

Spinal manipulation is one way to manage back pain without surgery.

Spinal manipulation, or chiropractic manipulation, involves using the hands to adjust, massage, or stimulate the spine.

In Kaushik Acupuncture, we have treated many patients with spinal manipulation for low back pain.

2. Acupuncture

Acupuncture is a Traditional Chinese Medicine practice. An acupuncture practitioner inserts thin needles into specific points on the body. WHO recommends acupuncture in above 28 chronic ailments including back pain. Kaushik Acupuncture offers one week program for back ache issues.

3. Weight Management

The back muscles, bones, and joints work hard to support the body as a person moves, sits, and stands. Being overweight can cause back pain due to increased pressure on the spine and strain of the back muscles. One study found that obesity has links to high levels of low back pain and disability. An ideal weight may help alleviate pain.

4. Anti-inflammatory diet

Higher levels of inflammation have a close connection to certain types of chronic pain. One way to help lower inflammation in the body is to follow an anti-inflammatory diet including vegetables, fruits, nuts, whole grains etc. Avoid processed food, fried items, sugars as they cause inflammation.

5. Correcting posture is most important

Having a good posture may help reduce back pain.

Incorrect posture could be the cause of back pain for some people, so taking steps to correct it may bring relief. Keep yourself in posture especially those with desk job and students.

6. Exercise

Although a person may find being active difficult when they are living with pain, movement is one of the best natural treatments for many types of pain.

Studies have long supported the fact that exercise can release endorphins which are body's natural pain killers. These natural brain chemicals help stop pain by binding to opioid receptors in the brain. This has a mild effect similar to opioid pain medications.

Research suggests that exercises that strengthen the back and neck muscles can reduce pain in people with chronic back and neck pain. Yoga and Breathing exercises are very useful but they should be done under supervision.

7. Proper footwear

Wearing the wrong type of footwear can cause the legs, hips, and back to misalign. This misalignment can lead to back pain. High heels, shoes that are too tight, or shoes that offer poor support are possible back pain culprits.

Dr. Kaushik's Recommendation for High Blood Pressure

If you are experiencing high blood pressure for a long time or have noticed high blood pressure recently, do not panic and take the following steps to get to the normal blood pressure.

We have been helped hundreds of patients through acupuncture and natural therapies with excellent results. These treatments are good for preventing as well as managing BP.

Dr Kaushik's Recommendation for High BP:

1. Throw sedentary lifestyle out of your life and be active.
2. Remove idealistic attitude from your life, take life at ease without hurry. Develop let go attitude. Control your emotional attitude like anger, fear, frustration through let go attitude, meditation and focused goal in life.
3. For cooking use oil free recipe and avoid packaged food, sweets, oil in any form. Avoid packaged and processed food and ban outside food. Eat wholesome food including Dalia, sprouts which give sufficient roughage. Minimize salt intake. Avoid fried irrespective of any oil.
4. Drink few glasses of lukewarm water first thing in the morning and half glass of water before going to bed.
5. Breakfast before 9 am with fruits (No juices).Most important meal to avoid BP.
6. Lunch by 1.30 pm with buttermilk and salads.
7. Dinner by 6.30 with soups, vegetables, no protein like pulses or non-veg in dinner.
8. Avoid smoking,
9. Restrict drinking to moderate level and it is always better to leave it.

10. Do yoga and meditation to avoid stress, the root cause of BP. Meditation especially transcendental meditation can normalize your BP just after 15-20 sessions.
11. Get acupuncture treatment for BP.
12. 20 minutes of a brisk walk in the morning and ten minutes of the walk after dinner.

13. Take 7 hours of sleep.
14. Keep your body alkaline.
15. Help others, enjoy community living which help if reducing stress to a significant level.
16. Be optimistic, try to find positive even out of negative incident. See one bad news can make you a BP patient and age your body 10 years faster, so even in a bad situation, learn to keep calm and have a belief that this situation will be over soon and a new beginning is waiting ahead.
17. Press P6 acupressure point and third eye acupressure points 2 minutes each daily.

Dr. Kaushik's recommendation for Cervical Spondylosis

Cervical spondylosis is a general term for age-related wear and tear affecting the spinal disks in your neck. As the disks dehydrate and shrink, signs of osteoarthritis develop, including bony projections along the edges of bones (bone spurs).

Cervical spondylosis is very common and worsens with age. More than 85 percent of people older than age 60 are affected by cervical spondylosis.

Most people experience no symptoms from these problems. When symptoms do occur, nonsurgical treatments like acupuncture and chiropractic are often are effective.

Dr Kaushik's recommendation for Cervical Spondylosis:

1. First of all improve your sitting posture with straight spine and do not put pressure on neck back while sitting. Take care specially during reading and working on computer.
2. Do not bend forward and avoid sudden posture change, do not sit in one posture for a long time. Take neck stretching exercises 3 times a day to strengthen the neck.
3. Optimize intake of calcium and magnesium, also take vitamin B6 and vitamin C after consulting your doctor.
4. To reduce pain do the following: Apply ice pack at the pain site for 20 minutes there after apply hot water bottle at the same place for same duration. After that apply tiger oil at the pain site and massage very gently for 5 minutes.
5. Avoid Yoga and exercise during pain and take rest.
6. Do yoga and meditation to avoid recurrence but under strict supervision.
7. Get acupuncture treatment and Chirpractic treatment , the best way to control neck problems.

Dr. Kaushik's Recommendation for Heart and good health

Preventing heart problem and keeping a young and healthy heart is first priority for everyone.

We have been treating heart patients through acupuncture and natural therapies with excellent results. These treatments are important for preventing a heart problem and if it has occurred then to avoid recurrence of the same.

Dr Kaushik's recommendation for a healthy heart:

1. Throw sedentary lifestyle out of your life and be active. Animals do not suffer from heart attack as they do not have sedentary lifestyle and are close to nature. Adopt a disciplined lifestyle.
2. Remove idealistic attitude from your life, take life at ease without hurry. Develop let go attitude.
3. For cooking use oil free recipe and avoid packaged food, sweets, oil in any form. Avoid packaged and processed food and ban outside food. Eat wholesome food including Dalia, sprouts which give sufficient roughage.
4. Drink four glasses of lukewarm water first thing in the morning and half glass of water before going to bed.
5. Breakfast before 9 am with fruits (No juices).
6. Lunch by 1.30 pm with buttermilk and salads.
7. Dinner by 6.30 with soups, vegetables, no protein like pulses or non-veg in dinner.
8. Avoid smoking, Drinking
9. Get health checkup twice a year.
10. Moderate exercise for 150 minutes a week is a must.
11. Do yoga and meditation to avoid stress, the root cause of heart problems.
12. Get one-week acupuncture treatment for heart care.
13. 20 minutes of a brisk walk in the morning and ten minutes of the walk after dinner.
14. Take 7 hours of sleep.
15. Keep check on BP and diabetes.

16. If possible take oil massage once in a month which helps in balancing vaat which is the cause of heart problem.
17. Keep your body alkaline. Heart attack is possible only in an acidic body and if you keep your body alkaline, you will never have a heart attack.
18. Minimize Acidic food : Meat, poultry, fish, dairy, eggs, grains and alcohol. Neutral: Natural fats, starches and sugars. Maximize Alkaline food: Fruits, nuts, legumes and vegetables.

Dr. Kaushik's Recommendation for Rheumatoid Arthritis (RA)

What is Rheumatoid Arthritis

Rheumatoid arthritis (RA) is the most common type of autoimmune arthritis. It is caused when the immune system (the body's defense system) is not working properly. RA causes pain and swelling in the wrist and small joints of the hand and feet. Treatments for RA can stop joint pain and swelling.

Diagnosis

Rheumatoid arthritis can be difficult to diagnose in its early stages because the early signs and symptoms mimic those of many other diseases. There is no one blood test or physical finding to confirm the diagnosis.

During the physical exam, your doctor will check your joints for swelling, redness and warmth. He or she may also check your reflexes and muscle strength.

Blood tests

People with rheumatoid arthritis often have an elevated erythrocyte sedimentation rate (ESR) or C-reactive protein (CRP), which may indicate the presence of an inflammatory process in the body. Other common blood tests look for rheumatoid factor and anti-cyclic citrullinated peptide (anti-CCP) antibodies.

Imaging tests

Your doctor may recommend X-rays to help track the progression of rheumatoid arthritis in your joints over time. MRI and ultrasound tests can help your doctor judge the severity of the disease in your body.

Dr Kaushik's recommendation for Rheumatoid Arthritis: Also helpful in Osteoarthritis

1. Look for the cause of inflammation in the joints which causes pain and swelling which may be due to weather change, wrong food etc. Remove the cause and you will get immediate relief.
2. Throw sedentary lifestyle out of your life and be active. Keep your joints moving, do some joint exercises.
3. Avoid sour and spicy food as they cause inflammation. Use freshly made food but do not use raw food, instead use freshly cooked food.
4. Drink few glasses of lukewarm water first thing in the morning and half glass of water before going to bed.
5. Breakfast before 9 am with fruits (No juices).
6. Lunch by 1.30 pm
7. Dinner by 6.30 with soups, vegetables, no protein like pulses or non-veg in dinner.
8. Avoid smoking, Drinking
9. Optimize intake of proteins but do not exceed required quantity.

10 Do yoga and meditation to avoid joint inflammation.

Dr. Kaushik's Recommendaton for Sciatica Pain

Sciatica refers to pain that radiates along the path of the sciatic nerve, which branches from your lower back through your hips and buttocks and down each leg. Typically, sciatica affects only one side of your body.

Sciatica most commonly occurs when a herniated disk, bone spur on the spine or narrowing of the spine (spinal stenosis) compresses part of the nerve. This causes inflammation, pain and often some numbness in the affected leg.

Although the pain associated with sciatica can be severe, most cases resolve with non-operative treatments in a few weeks. People who have severe sciatica that's associated with significant leg weakness or bowel or bladder changes might require immediate attention.

Dr Kaushik's recommendation for Sciatica Pain:

1. First of all improve your sitting posture with straight spine and do not put pressure on lower back while sitting.
2.   Do not bend forward and avoid sudden posture change, do not sit in one posture for a long time.
3. Optimize intake of calcium and magnesium regularly, also take vitamin B6 and vitamin C as per doctor advise.
4. To reduce pain do the following:

    Apply ice pack at the pain site for 10 minutes, there after apply hot water bottle at the same place for same duration.

    After that apply tiger oil at the pain site and massage very gently for 5 minutes.

    Avoid lifting weight during pain.

5. Avoid Yoga and exercise during pain and take rest.

6. Do yoga and meditation to avoid recurrence but under strict supervision.
7. Get one-week acupuncture treatment and Chiropractic treatment.

Five Ayurvedic eating habits for a healthier ageing

There are many different habit changes you can incorporate into your lifestyle which will benefit your health and wellbeing. Here are five ayurvedic and natural habits that can help you live a healthier Life.

- 1- In a world full of excess it is better to keep meals to one or two times a day. The three meals a day plus all the snacking and social eating is one of the major cause of lifestyle diseases in modern society. This tradition of breakfast, lunch and dinner is not very modern any more. You should eat when you need food and not because it is 'time to eat.' How can it be time to eat for every single person at the same time? A healthy mind and body only needs 1 to 2 meals a day and that is without snacks. Some days the body also needs a complete rest from intake of food, therefore a fast of warm water is recommended. Fasting has great importance in naturopathy and Ayurvedic practice.

- 2 - The timing of eating is crucial and this needs to be way before bedtime so the body has a chance to do some cleaning during the night. Eating before 5 or 6pm is a health habit to cultivate. This will give the system time to digest the food and then when you are sleeping no energy needs to be wasted on digestion and at the same time no extra toxins are created from undigested food passing into the intestines.

- 3 - Eating in season is fundamental to a healthy diet. A local farmers market is best as they have local produce which is in season and your body is acclimated to that type of food. Eating foods that are brought in from all over the world creates many issues such as allergies, digestive problems, skin toxicity and constipation. Eat local fresh foods and avoid problems.

- 4 - Eat in the right combinations of foods. Eating in season alleviates much of this problem but then there are many other foods which should not be mixed together.

- 5 - Fill the stomach with two third foods and leave one third empty. As you leave room for digestion food digestion becomes easy and your food is digested properly leaving very little room for toxic formation. This rule will change if a person is very imbalanced in one element or another but in general this is a good guide line for a healthy food intake.

18 forever according to Chinese Medicine

In today's developed and medically advanced world, we are aging fast and are catching up life threatening diseases and chronic diseases at a very early stage because of decreased immunity and resistance to disease. When we talk of aging, we talk of biological age and not the chronological one. When you see a 60 year old woman and says… wow, she looks only 30 and on the other side a 30 year old looks like 60. This can be achieved by countering stress and life events by improving your overall stamina and by eliminating the root cause of the aging and chronic diseases. Let us understand the causes of fast aging and chronic ailments. The answer to this lies in Chinese medicine. There are two types of energies in all living beings, pre-birth energy or Qi and post-birth energy or Qi. The way we age and become prone to chronic ailments is affected by both our parents at the time of conception and on future mother during pregnancy and this we cannot change. But post birth Qi or energy also decides how we age and most of this Qi depends on our lifestyle. Post birth energy or Qi can be enhanced and maintained with good diet, regular exercise, good sleep, enjoying life and having fun, avoiding stress, handling negative emotions like anger and staying away from addictive substances. But what we can not control are our life events such as sudden bad news like death of a near one or a traumatic accident which can age us 10 years over night or can affect our brain and body. Life events specially the negative one are the root cause of the aggravated emotions like anger, grief and fear which damages our brain and we age fast. The best way to control the damage caused by bad events is to meditate on regular basis and adopt drugless healing therapies and say no to all types of drugs. And I have done this with thousands of my patients. This will help you in making mind and body strong enough to counter life challenges including lifestyle diseases. And last but not the least , feel young and feel 18 till you die.

The Secret of Living Well and Longer Is Eat Half, Walk Double, Laugh Triple and Love Without Measure.

-Tibetan Proverb

Constipation solution as per Acupuncture & TCM

In eastern Medicine, constipation is a medical problem and is considered as root cause of many other chronic diseases. Every second person face this problem. I do not prefer drugs to control constipation and advise natural way to deal with it.

Chronic constipation causes:

lack of hydration or lubrication,

not enough exercise,

not enough fiber.

But also emotional stress, holding on to something (the large intestine is the organ that let go!).

Self-treatment options:

- A glass of warm water with sea salt.

- Eating more seeds & nuts, avocado, cucumber, tomato, fruits, veggies, broth. Prunes!

- Massaging the belly in circles clockwise (following the large intestine path).

- Eat less refined food and if possible maintain fix timings.

- Eat food with more and more fiber.

- 10 to 12 glasses of water every day.

- Avoid overthinking as it causes constipation, if possible meditate.

Managing Autoimmune Diseases with Acupuncture and Diet

Autoimmune disease happens when the body's natural defense system can't tell the difference between your own cells and foreign cells, causing the body to mistakenly attack normal cells. There are more than 80 types of autoimmune diseases that affect a wide range of body parts.

Autoimmune diseases are increasingly common. Millions of Indians are suffering from a least one kind of auto-immune disorder. If you have an autoimmune disease, it means that your body is basically attacking itself. Your immune system goes into overdrive and sees everything as a threat. Trying to protect you from this perceived danger, it starts fighting and attacking its own tissues and cells, mistaking them as hazards. This can lead to pain, discomfort, and all kinds of issues depending on the autoimmune condition you have.

Despite the wide range of different autoimmune diseases though, they all tend to have the same kinds of triggers. If you avoid these common triggers, you can avoid flare-ups and reduce your symptoms.

Autoimmune Disease Triggers

Genetics: Certain disorders such as lupus and multiple sclerosis (MS) tend to run in families. Having a relative with autoimmune disease increases your risk, but it doesn't mean you will develop a disease for certain.

Weight: Being overweight or obese raises your risk of developing rheumatoid arthritis or psoriatic arthritis. This could be because more weight puts greater stress on the joints or because fat tissue makes substances that encourage inflammation.

Smoking: Research has linked smoking to a number of autoimmune diseases, including lupus, rheumatoid arthritis, hyperthyroidism and MS.

Sugar:

Processed sugar is a common offender for anyone's health. It leads to inflammation and can trigger autoimmune symptoms. Use organic honey and eat dates, fruits, and root veggies for sweetness.

Quinoa.

Though it is gluten-free and a trendy protein-rich pseudo grain, in large amounts, it can actually provoke your immune system. Limit your quinoa consumption and stick to other gluten-free products instead.

Gluten.

Gluten is a well-known offender of health. People with Celiac disease know to stay away from it, however, it is destructive to anyone with any other autoimmune condition as well. Switch to gluten-free to stay safe.

Dairy.

Due to molecular mimicry, casein in dairy can act like gluten in your body. It can cause your immune system to go haywire and trigger your symptoms. Switch to plant-based alternatives. If you need sweetness, fruit and root veggies are your best options.

If you avoid these triggers, you can reduce your risks of an autoimmuneflare-up.

ACUPUNCTURE AND OTHER NATURAL MEDICINE OPTIONS CAN HELP IN MANAGING YOUR CONDITION. We have used alternative medicine as an option to manage autoimmune disorders by controlling inflammation and pain.